Healing Pilates

I0421096

Successful Guide to Pilates Anatomy Pilates Exercises and Total Body Fitness

SECOND EDITION

By Ellena Ivanov

Contents

Introduction

There are many exercise systems that exist in the world today, and it is essential that you identify one that will work for you and your body. A holistic solution is best, allowing you to attain weight loss, as well as strengthen and tone your muscles.

Pilates is a system of exercise that is holistic in nature. It was developed by Joseph Pilates in the early 1900s and since it has been practiced, has increased in popularity and is now carried out by people from all over the world. The exercises that are done in Pilates are designed to strengthen the muscles in the body, improve the overall flexibility of the person, and essentially build up one's overall health.

Today, Pilates is also an excellent way to lose weight and stay in shape, as it can be practiced by any person, no matter what they level of fitness, age or walk of life. This eBook contains all the information that you will need to know about Pilates, and how it is that you can get started.

You will find out what it actually entails, and the many benefits this system of exercise will have on your health. There is also information on how to choose an instructor that will help you meet your ultimate weight loss and fitness goals. In addition, there are detailed exercises for you to try, so that if you want to immediately begin working on Pilates, you can do so with this book.

Essentially, this book is your go to guide that offers you a complete solution on everything to do with Pilates. Read on and change the way that you look at fitness, starting now.

Chapter 1:
The Need For Body Trimming

None of us can deny the pressures on our souls because of these fast moving life patterns. All day long, we move from one place to another, for working deadlines, household chores and special agreements. This has made the human life more liable towards robotic routines. Every rising sun is having some different and variant challenge. Many people owe this extensive development and progress of mankind in the field of technology and research. As more and more aspects are being conquered, the challenges for humans are also becoming gigantic. Therefore, in this tiresome war of survival, the human beings have nearly forgotten their existence and the need for taking care of one's self.

Apart from various needs like those that the physiological and the need for accomplishment, there have are innumerable reasons, which can be listed for making the human posture fit and trim.

The tiresome routines

As discussed in the introductory notes, human life is no less than a challenge. In this venture of financial struggle, many of us have become ignorant for their individualistic needs. Spending hours and hours sitting on our workstations, in a need to earn more and to get prominent position in one's corporate and social circle, we have left our self far away. Other than physical fatigue, all this tiresome challenge has posed a number of questions for the quality of life. While planning our lives, we should account for a balanced approach, an approach that can aid us in meeting the both ends. One major thing which needs to be accounted for is the dependency of this entire struggle on human health. So while on our way to challenging work life, we should also keep an eye on the need for keeping our body slim and trim.

The decreased immunity level

As all pictures having two side of analysis, the technology outburst has also given birth to a number of major aftermaths pertaining to human life. All these points are interconnected. The demanding routine of work has made individuals less concerned towards their body needs. As a result the dependency over processed and easy to eat food has increased to a horrible level. All the artificial food and processed diet patterns has made the human body internally weak, so much so that the munity level against the infections and bacterial attacks has reduced to an alarming level.

Reliance on technology big cut to physical activity

Yet another aftermath of this technology dependent human world has been observed in the shape of reduced physical activity. We have become surrounded by machines, robots and digital assistants. Form mobile phone to large space rockets all the inventions of technology has drastically altered the human routine. The increased dependency on machines has led to extremely low levels of physical activities. So the human body has become addict of no physical output. All work is done through workstations, with just a few clicks. From shopping to planning everything is mechanized form ordering to online delivery. All this has put human far from physical activity and more inclined towards obesity and health issues.

Overweight denotes social humiliation

Connecting all these major points ne major consequence is the increased trend of obesity and being overweight. The story does not end here. In fact it is the commencement of a new quandary. Because of having a detracted body, many of us have to encounter blunt remarks and humiliating statements. It is a severe trauma for the individual suffering from it, as he has a sturdy routine, and is not equipped to spend any of his time for his body trimming. The situation become even worse if re affected individual is a female. Female being highly possessive about body shape and beauty become extremely fatigued about this matter, the social mortification faced by being overweight leads towards the mental and emotional disturbances. So the need for body trimming has heightened greatly.

Chapter 2:
The Emergence of Pilates- Setting Miraculous Standards for Human World

Pilates is a term used for an exclusive classification of strengthening, stabilizing and stretching exercises, introduced about ninety years ago by Joseph H. Pilates, who was basically a German born. He was a physical culturist. The history of his upbringing strongly connotes his interest n the field of physical arts, as his mother was a naturopath and his father worked for long as a gymnast. His father won a number of prizes and distinction in this filed. Being brought up in such an environment, Pilates naturally had the tendency to get interested in physical arts and exercises. He learned and practiced varying categories of exercise including yoga, both Eastern trends as well as the Western forms of exercise.

Earlier in his youth, he was skillful in a number of physical training regimes, which were practiced at that time in Germany. All this summed up for his inspiration for developing the idea of Pilates. These were the time traced back to late ninetieth century when the physical culture was taking a turn and the use of exercises as a preventive as well as a curative technique, was gaining momentum. One f the result of these changed trends was the use of apparatuses. An additional and chief whirling point in his career was the war time. At that time he got trapped in Britain because of war. During that time medical gymnastics emerged as a popular trend. Joseph Pilates also started instructing corrective exercise.

The theme line of Pilates as a fitness instrument is that the powerhouse of human body is the center of the human body. So this technique is exclusively focuses on the postural muscles, to regain a perfect posture. The apparatus used in different sessions, the Allegro Reformer, uses straps, springs, and a stirring carriage to provide for a variety of exercises and to create spatial and body awareness. Pilates is a scheme for attaining the body awareness. Having a firm belief in and having the determination to get results with Pilate's scheme will revolutionize your entire life, the mode of your feeling your own appearance will change altogether

Return to Life through Contrology

Joseph H. Pilates spent a major portion of his life in United States a and made major developments upon his research work there, Therefore United States became the major hub for the progress and popularity of this technique. It is largely being followed in the United States

Although the technique has become renowned all over the world as "Pilates" because of the unprecedented contribution of its inventor, yet the original term coined by the pioneer was Contrology, from the combination of control and logia (being of Greek origin)

In his book Joseph Pilates proposed that this scheme of exercise is basically an art of highly controlled and calculate movements, which, when properly administrated, will have a feeling of a workout, rather than some imposed kind of therapy. owed to constant practicing Pilates retains the ability to aid in getting flexibility, control, strength, develops control and endurance in the entire body and posture. It entails a prominence to breathing, alignment, coordination, and development of a strapping powerhouse and balance. This

6

scheme of exercise brings out for different exercises to be adapted in a variant range of toughness, from commencement to complex or to any other level. The exercise pattern may also alter or vary depending on the personalized goals of practitioner and the choice of instructors.

Pilates had a strong belief that mental strength and physical health are highly and critically dependant o one another.

The mechanical aspects of "Pilates

Joseph Pilates being the inventor of this technique was not only a gymnast. he was also a scientist as well as a, mechanical genius This aided him o accompany his method by a set of useful equipments which he denoted as "apparatus" .The Apparatus acted as an aid to help pick up the pace or the entire process of <u>body alignment</u>, <u>strengthening</u>, <u>stretching</u>, and increased core strength. The best-known and most popular piece today, Reformer, was in the beginning designated as the Universal Reformer, rightly designated for reforming the body universally. As more and more progress HAS Underwent in the flied of Pilates, there has developed a full array of accessories and equipments. This includes the Pedi-Pole, Wunda Chair, Cadillac, High "Electric" Chair, Ladder Barrel and Spine Corrector.

Publications of Joseph Pilates:

- Your Health: A Corrective System of Exercising (1934)

- Return to Life Through Contrology (1945)

Modern Pilates embraces both the traditional approach of Pilates, as well as the modern additions in the scheme. The classical approach to Pilates is based on the original and unedited work of Joseph Pilates, the legend; whereas the current versions are based on slight alterations and modifications, made mostly by first generation students. But most of the people are of the view that this mixture of new and old has largely benefited the field and it has expanded the scope of Pilates from being a mere exercise to a whole therapeutic approach. So this addition has benefited a lot for all the practitioners, in various fields, and also put great emphasis for the need of physical health.

At the time when it was first introduced, Pilates technique was confined to specialized surroundings like studios and Pilates center, but as the benefits of Pilates have outburst at an exponential rate, the facility has now been adopted by various gyms, exercise centers and physiotherapy rooms .The major reason for this diversity in the available spaces for Pilates, can easily be accounted for its highly influential effects and far reaching benefits. Many of the physical instructors are modifying this technique along with their own ways of exercise and physical art. This has made the field of Pilates, a greatly enriched field, in which every new day brings a lot of diversity and new techniques. All over the world people now consider it as more of a therapeutic technique, which is bestowing health and rigor all over the world to millions of people who were hopeless after some ailment or their distorted body type.

Chapter 3:
The Astounding Effects of Pilates

Fitness is the first mandatory for contentment and joy. A common belief about the nature of physical fitness is the accomplishment and continuation of a consistently maintained body with an active mind, which entails the capability of undergoing all tasks with promptness and diligence. To attain the premier success, within the boundaries of one's capacities, in all domains and arenas of life, the preceding significance must be given to get healthier and developed body systems. Once physical rigor is established, it will without human intervention overlay the system towards mental zest and intelligence.

But all this is easy to write and say. Once you start implementing this, you will find a lot many hindrances. Among the supreme challenges is to keep streamlined while being in this challenging world, where everything is hard to achieve. The work pressures, the family demands and the individual needs, all sum up to make the life more messy and challenging. In all this one forgets to think and hover upon his own individual being. Most f the time we think that the last priority we think of, is ourselves. We assume it wrongly that our responsibility is to thrive in all fields of life, leaving behind all necessities of our own health. But in this busy scheduled life, we forget that vigor is foreseeable and remote, despite of all financial resources. Once gone, health needs excessive efforts to be restored.

Physical fitness is both a dilemma and a blessing. It is a kind of state which can never be achieved through heavy investments or by ere thinking. It demands for full exertion and efforts. The results are always twofold. Higher the rate of exertion, definitely higher will be the benefits achieved. But the modern system of human civilization has ruined this need of human being, by engaging it in a number of irrelevant and disastrous tasks, including increased reliance on technology and robotic inventions. Although fiscally one may be mountaineering the ladders of triumph, but the health arena of one's life may fall insolvent. So balancing both sides of the pivot is the key for life, eventually one can be labeled as the real victorious person. If an individual is quite successful in the work life, but he has ruined his health and body, he cannot be labeled as a successful man because he has opted for one, among the two most crucial aspects of life,

Among all these panics and challenges, Pilates has emerged as a major revolutionary step. Among a number of different useful aspects of Pilates, some of them are reflected and discussed below:

For weight loss:

One of the major disasters created by this challenging life is the life routines which ultimately make the human body fatty and overweight. Overweight induces a number of various physical issues which can retain for longer periods, ultimately leading to disasters in human health. Pilates is miraculous for weight loss. The systematic procedures and techniques of Pilates lead towards burning of fat that will assist in making the body slimmed and trimmed, within no time. But the key to triumph is the consistency in the routines and practicing of Pilates. This scheme of body exercise help you monitor your body, modify your breathing patterns, so that all these functions of human body can be changed into an efficient and highly effective body system. Most of the Pilates schemes which are aimed for body weight loss denote the stretching exercises.

For dancers

Pilates is not only for curative purposes, meaning that it is not only a technique for the curative purposes. It is not for all those who have ruined their body postures and shape, it can also help a lot many who are involved in a number of stretching professions or other activities which involve excessive physical outputs. Among these professionals, one of the largest groups involves dancers. Dancers are therapists who use their body language to convey their art. They cannot afford even a minimum sort of body disturbances. Moreover, a number of Pilate's techniques involve the postures which ultimately lead to highly flexible body organs, so it aid in using the body more effectively by the dancers. Various dancers have reported that they have experienced a wide appreciation because of changed body reflexive due to Pilates.

During pregnancy

Many women think that they are cannot exert much physical efforts if they have got pregnant. Pregnancy does not denote physical statistic. It must be accompanied with healthy routines and living patterns. Pilates is a distinctive workout scheme which can pose a number of techniques for pregnant ladies, which will not only lend a hand to them for retaining their body shapes but will also aid in progressive development of the baby's body. Although pregnancy needs excessive monitoring for body, yet it does not demand that all the physical activity must be stopped immediately after getting the good news. The whole period of pregnancy must be engaged in a way that it becomes productive for the health and physique, not a burden. Pilates introduces some basic regimes of body and leg movement for all ladies who are having these issues and help them cater their pregnancy in a better way. If the women start it form the initial stage to last stage she will definitely enjoy an overwhelmingly secure and sound pregnancy without any complications.

For belly fat

Some specific issues addressed by Pilates also include the belly fat issues. Any excessive fat deposit or lipoid-deposit is easily manageable by some modified techniques of Pilates, which help in calorie burning and fat dissolution. Many of the thinkers hold the analysis that belly fat reduction demands for a consistent approach towards following a regular scheme. Belly fat reduction is considered as one of the major challenges as well as a hindrance towards slim and trim body. Many of the Pilates techniques have been specially modified, to help a large number of people, who are facing a downturn in their body. The reason for this downturn is the increased fat on their belly. It also hits the body and the personality charisma. No one likes to be recognized by a loose tummy. So Pilates can help everyone start an energetic and charismatic life by trimming the belly and making all the muscles healthy strong and still attractive.

For back pain

One of the key reasons for back ache is the distorted body postures. These postures are usually induced by unhealthy sitting postures and uncomfortable sitting plan. Moreover back pain can be because of higher tendency towards obesity and the tendency of being overweight. All these basic reasons can contribute towards the highly painful condition of back ache. Pilates is aimed at not only curing back ache nut also preventing it in all those, who have not encountered it. The stretching exercises and the postures introduced by Pilates help in strengthen of spinal cord and the vertebrae so that it can maintain the back strength and avoid all the reasons effectively. Back ache has been reported to be one of the major reasons of distorted body shapes, so eradicating it form the basic level is highly crucial.

For abs

Another misconception about Pilate's method is that it is only a way of correcting the posture, body movements and breathing patterns. Many people are devoid of the information that Pilates is also for all those who want to build up a muscular body. Abs building is another miracle of Pilate's scheme of exercise. Although the scheme and pattern of exercise will be quite transformed for abs building, yet Pilates is not devoid of these kinds of techniques which are helpful for body builders and all those who are interested in muscle formation. Many people have been successful in building and sustain their abs because they have consistently followed Pilate's scheme.

For strength

Pilates is an excellent way of helping your body improve on its overall strength. When you go to the gym, you often work out your muscles by isolating them so that you can build some bulk in particular muscle in your body. With Pilates, you are able to work on every single muscle in your body, as the movements connect all of these muscles together. Pilates can be viewed as exercise that places emphases on the strengthening of the entire body through stretching and working the muscles. At the end of your Pilates sessions, you would have succeeded in strengthening your body without having the worry of adding bulk as would be expected from someone who is going to the gym for the same.

For aesthetics

Most people will work out because they are looking to get an excellent body which they love to look at and that other people can admire as well. Pilates helps you to accomplish this for your own body. This is because it features both oppositional and correctional movements, which changes the way that muscles behave and react. In a short period doing Pilates, the muscles on your body will begin to change shape and you will have better definition that is graceful. This will help you look stronger and healthier, without making you look bulky and "pumped up". The parts of your body that will see the most benefit from Pilates include your stomach or abdomen, your bottom and your thighs and legs.

For posture

For people who are having any types of issues with their posture, Pilates offers and excellent solution, allowing them to ideally strengthen their posture in various ways. This is because the exercises that you will execute in Pilates demand for one to be able to balance themselves well and maintain an excellent posture at all times. After several sessions of Pilates you will find that you stand up straighter and have less of an imbalance in your body. This is exercise that is appropriate for people of all ages, so if you have a child whose posture you would like to improve on as well, practicing Pilates is key.

For better sleep

Pilates is ideal for you to try if you are looking for any way to overcome your insomnia. It allows you to wind down, and for your body to be relaxed enough to ensure that your nervous system helps you to get the rest you need. By doing Pilates, particularly the rolling and unrolling exercise, you are in effect giving your spine a massage and reliving your nerves from build up pressure. Increasing your flexibility and helping cleanse your body through exercise makes it easier for you to relax and get a good night's sleep. There are even some Pilates exercises that you can try out in bed so that you accomplish better sleep.

For a better sex life

Pilates helps to relax your muscles and increase your flexibility. You will find that many times your sex life may be hindered because of a lack of confidence about how your body works and moves. By introducing Pilates into your life, you are essentially changing the way your body moves. The breathing exercises that you do will help you to become more present, and the fact that Pilates also has an effect on the body and what it looks like means that your confidence will be considerably increased.

For everyone

Pilates can be done by everyone. It is ideal to be practiced by men who are athletic as it will help them to find balance in their bodies. For women of all ages, it can help restore flexibility and increase core strength. For children, it helps with correcting issues that have to do with balance, and also with maintaining good posture. It is an excellent holistic exercise system which can be adequately exploited to bring about brilliant benefits.

Chapter 4:
Starting With Pilates

Pilates or as proposed by its inventor, Contrology is an absolute synchronization and dexterity of soul, mind and body. In the course of learning and practicing Pilates the practitioners first decisively obtain an efficient control over all the body movements and functions and this control and management is then utilized to acquire the synchronization of soul and subconscious activities. When all the different domains of the body and soul are following the same synchronization and harmony, the eventual result will be the healthy and peaceful body.

But all this harmonization and management requires consistency and the sense of determination so that repetitive Pilates practicing can lead you to achieve your desired goals.

Pilates is the most renowned and effective technique for correcting imbalanced body postures, developing body health, enhancing the spirits and restoring the physical vivacity. These characteristics are basically inbuilt in the human body, when the humans are in the early age of infancy, when soul and body directions are same, coherent and efficient. But this purity and synchronization is soon lost when the infant steadily moves toward maturity and start facing the harsh and cruel realities of life. During this course of challenging battle with the realities of life, the first thing that gets hurt is the physical attire of the human body. The aftermaths can be experiential in the shape of fatigued eyes, callous crows' feet, spun out shoulders and indistinct postures. Many people consider it to be the aftermaths of growing age but this is not true because growing age does not connotes bad health. All we need is to restore the vitality and rigor of our body and taking care of our soul and busy as some precious treasure, upon which the whole essence of our success relies. Pilates is among some techniques which help you revitalize your body muscles and strengths.

Principles of Pilates:

Although we can have been discussing what the field of Pilates technique for body stability has become such a diverse field that different sort of modifications, alterations and additions have made it more useful technique, yet some basics of Pilates involves the core themes of principles of this techniques.

Concentration

The core is to concentrate. Many of you may ask that when we are overwhelmed with so much of work pressures and deadlines that getting in the stream of focus is quite near to impossible. So Pilate's techniques help you to develop and craft the ability to concentrate. Concentration is vital because Pilate's scheme of exercise is aimed at making the individual relieved form the worries and pressures, so by developing concentration these exercises can easily let the practitioner get away from the worries and concentration the workout. The actual results of this technique are also visible when the stage of concentration becomes achievable.

Control

Control denotes the power of managing the body movements, muscular strengths and body patterns. Although these principles are the successive steps of Pilate's technique, yet they are highly interrelated. Concentration and excess of focus will eventually pave your way towards body control and management. Many of you may ponder upon the need for control. The basic theme of Pilates is to let everyone enjoy the manageability if ones, body movements and postures, so Pilates will help you learn this.

Centering

In Pilates scheme of exercise the focus on some initial point of reference or centering position. Most if the viewpoints regarding the center have made the central abdominal region as the main focus of the body movements and the point of management. Hence the entire scheme of abdominal muscles and the limbs are highly focused and maintained to serve as the center of strength and rigor.

Flow of movement

Once the control over the body is achieved than the trainers usually advice to start practicing the management of movements and dynamic systems of the body. The limbs are highly focused, so that the movements are according to the standards of efficient body which can correct the body postures and tart paving the way to vitalized body. Once the body movements are managed they will become the part of human routines and working style so that physical stress cannot destroy the human health.

Precision

Accuracy is the critical and crucial factor. The entire the activities and posters experienced in that scheme of study are designed with zero error precision, as human body is also prone to is management. Although human body denotes strength and rigor yet it can be fragile if exposed to mismanaged body postures and movements. So the instructors of Pilates usually take care of this aspect and design every exercise according individual inclinations and abilities. A slight ignorance from the individual needs of the human body can drastically destroy the precision of the exercise and the fruitful results of the exercise can never be accounted. Precision looks very irrelevant to common man as far as the physical output is considered, yet it lies as the main foundation of Pilates.

Breathing

Apart from body movements the basics of human body control is the pattern of breathing. One trivial amendment and improvement in breathing patterns and techniques can help the human body enjoy the maximum of power and vitality. Pilate's instructor helps individuals use this function of human body as the source of power. Individuals are taught t breath with efficient styles and using different routes, which also varies according to individual objectives. Many of the latent faulty working and diseases of the human body can easily be eradicated if the breathing is considered not only as the function of human body but also strength for gaining the ultimate vitality and health.

Power house

Another distinctive characteristic of this scheme of physical exercise and output is the focus on the power house with reference to the human body as a system harmonized organs. As per the philosophy of Pilates the power house resides within the centre of human body. So all the basic principles focused above ultimately lead to the strengthening of this power house.

Chapter 5:
Why Choose Pilates?

There are so many other exercises that exist that promise to help you to tone your muscles and strengthen your body. After you have had a time to expereince or read up on some of them, why should you choose Pilates instead?

Here are some of the reasons that will bring Pilates to life for you.

Build Up the Whole Body

When you go to the gym, you may find that you work one part of your body more than the others.It is easy to work on your arms and build up your biceps and triceps, then find that you neglected your thighs and calves. This leads to you being out of proprootion, and worse, not happy with your body.

Pilates is one exercise that does not neglect any part of the body, and the reason for this is its focus on your core strength.

Everything begins with the core with Pilates, and so your body learns how to function as an entire unit, rather then just a prticular part. Overall strength is promoted, as is increased flexibility in the body. The point of Pilates is to build up your joints.

There is also the psychological aspect of development that you will find with Pilates. This is the effect of Pilates on your mind. One thing Pilates calls you to do is stop and focus on what you are doing and the exercises you are carrying out. You need to take long and deep breaths, which allows for your body and your mind to relax. This adds a dimension to fitness that other exercises might not provide.

Many Learning Methods

The best way to start off learning Pilates would be to go to a Pilates instructor and get some private lessons. By understanding you and your body, you can come up with exercises that will build your strength and increase your chances of success. What do you do if you do not have the means to get to an instructor, and still want to enjoy the benefits of Pilates?

This is one type of exercise that is easy to learn. You can attempt to teach yourself the techniques at your convience and in your own time. What you need to have is the right starting equipment and the proper attire.

All you need to begin with is a Pilates mat. From there, you can easily follow instructional videos that are available on the internet. You could also get some books and study the movements, like you will with this ebook. Pilates is not complicated, an dit is difficult for you to get it wrong.

For the Pilates Body

People who do Pilates have leaner bodies that are better aligned and beautifully toned. Working on the core of the body is an ideal way for a person to improve their breathing as well as their circulation. The techniques for breathing in Pilates help a person to slow down in what they are doing, and this in turn helps the circulatory system of the body. The Pilates body is not all about aethetics and looking good. There is the benefit of how it operates inside as well.

Blood circulation improves exponentially when one practices Pilates, as the blood gets detoxified from all the oxygen that it receives. This improves the natural rythmn from within, and refreshes the system.

Another added benefit is the strong spine which increases in flexibility as a result of the exercises. This is due to the core muscles offering support to the spine during the exercises, which in turn improves the alignment of all the bones within the body.

People with back pain will rave about the benefit they have experienced as a result of practicing Pilates for an extended period of time.

Chapter 6:
Choosing a Pilates Instructor

When you deide to being Pilates, it is best to start with an instructor who can show you the ropes and help you to learn all the basic techniques.It is essential that you choose an instructor who is familiar with all the systems of excecise in Pilates, because this type of workout iss based in scientific ptinciples. Your instructor should be able to both train you well, and to communicate with you an what needs to be done. The experience that you have as a student of Pilates will largely affect the level of success that you hope to attain.

This chapter contains some pointers that you should seek when looking for your ideal instructor.

Find out about Pilates

Pilates is not the sort of exercise where you go into the Pilates studio, have a short class and then head home. It is intense in nature and follows an in depth system for it to be effective. You will need to start off with a fixed number of sessions, and at the end of these sessions you will be in a position to tel whether the exercises are working for you or not.

For this reason, you need an instructor who is well qualified and expereinced in teaching Pilates. You should ensure that at a minimum, your instructor has 450 hours of comprehensive Pilates Instructor training.

Clarity of Instruction

You need to understand what your instructor is telling you so that you can carry out their instructions clearly. Before you make a final choice, attend one of their sessions and observe them. If you find that even by watching you are a little confused, then move on until you find someone whose communuication and instruction is clear for you.

Professionalism and Confidence

You will be working closely with your instructor, and therefore, you need to ensure that they are very professional in the way that they interact with you. Your instructor will have to touch you on occasion, and when this happens, you shuold never feel as if the instructor is being inappropriate. The best way to check on the level of professionalism is to speak to other students who are in the class and get a feel of how comfortable they are.

Enjoyable and Motivational

Your Pilates class is not torture exercise, and so at the end of it all it is expected that you had an enjoyable experience. Your instructor should help you feel as though what you are doing is fun. You also need to be motivated, and this can happen if your instructor checks in on you to ensure that the class is going as you expect, and also ensures that you are not experiencing any pain or discomfort in your body.

Meeting your Needs

Before you begin a session with your Pilates Instructor, it is important that time is taken to identify your needs and come up with a series of exercises that best suits you. Ensure that your instructor teaches the traditional Pilates as it was designed, as there are many new approached that have not yet been adequately tried and tested. You also need to have an instrcutor that is passionate and interested in helping you achieve your goals and this should be reflected by their actions

The Mind Should Be in Focus

Pilates is more than just a workout for the body, there is also the aspect of creating some balance in the mind. The instructor should be able to attain this type of balance by including some sort of moving meditation in the exercises that you will be performing. If you find that your instructor is only interested in testing out a range of proprs and taking you through loads of new exercises, you need to change them to someone who can better meet your needs.

Variety is Key

Everytime you go for a Pilates class, you should have some standard exercises that you do, and there should be something new. You should find yourself embroiled in a learning experience, and not in an experience that is focused on repetition and strict routine. Your instructr should be able to introduce new exercises to your seamlessly, so that you are not worried that you will plateau during your work out. If there are not too many new exercises being taught, there should at least be some variations to the older ones.

Certification

In line with being qualified to teach Pilates, your instructor should also be cetified by an accredited and recognised organisation. Just because someone has practical experience in trying out Pilates on their own, does not qualify them to be able to teach Pilates to others. You need someone who has a background in Pilates, and possible also has training in another type of movement such as yoga. Then you will get the best possible benefit for your body.

Chapter 7:
Practical Pilates – Preparing for Pilates Mat Exercises

Now that you know all about Pilates, it is right for you to try some if the exercises for your overall health, well being and weight management. You need to ensure that you are appropriately prepared, and this chapter will provide you with all the tools that you need to get your started.

It is likely that you will begin your expience with Pilates in a Pilates studio. Here, you will have the choice of two types of workouts. The first workout would require you to use a Pilates mat, and the second type of workout needs a Pilates apparatus. If you are a fresh beginner, it is advised that you begin with the Pilates mat, and once you have developed some skill, move on to use the Pilates apparatys.

Pilates Mat Classes are the best way to experience all the possible benefits hat you can get from Pilates. They are designed to be holistic in nature, and as you practice them you will find that you are toning your muscles, incresing your flexibility, as well as improving your posture. The connection between your mind and body will be strenthened. There is also the benefit of being able to do these exercises without relying on complicated aparatus to begin with.

Preparing for Pilates Mat Exercises

These are a series of exercises that any one can try, no matter what level of Pilates they have attained. You will practice all the basics and perfect them on the mat, and for your body, you have the added benefit of getting a significant amount of strength and also building your confidence in practicing Pilates.

If you are working out at a Pilates studio, you will find that it is equipped with mats. Should you opt to use one of these mats, it would be hygeinic for you to carry along a towel to cover it while you do the exercises. The more seasoned you become, the higher the likelihood that you will want to purchase and use your own mat for these exercises. These mats are easily available for purchase.

It is worth noting that the Pilates mat is usually thicker than the yoga mat, so it is not advisable to intercahnge them. With yoga, you do a considerable amount of exercises on your feet, and you need to have a better feel of the grouund beneath you. However, with Pilates, you are more likley to do exercises where you roll on your lower back, and you need the cushioning that the thicker mats can provide.They are available in a variety of colours, sizes and in different styles as well, so it will be possible to find one that meets your personal preferences.

You must also ensure that you are dressed in the appropriate gear for your Pilates workout. As your body will do plenty of stretching, you need to wear clothes that allow you to extend your flexibility. This ,eams that they should be stretchy, and allow for movement. They need to fit your body well, as the person who is instructing the class needs to see whether your muscles and bones are engaging as required. Therefore, leave your tracksuits and t-shirts out of this class.

You do not ened to have special shoes when doing Pilates mat exercises as for maximu effect, most of the mat exercises are done barefoot. If you are uncomfortable with being barefoot during the class, or are concerned that you could slip and hurt yourself, you can do the class while wearing a pair of socks for protection. Accessories should also be minimal or if possible left out entirely. This includes items that will dangle when you move such as bracelets and necklesses and big bulky rings that may affect the way you move your arms.

When it comes to your hair, the best option would be to have it tied back or pulled away from the face. In order for Pilates to be effective, you need to minimise the amount of distractions and all the causes of these distractions effectively.

At this point you are physically ready for the workout. To make sure that you can last the entire duration without worry, ensure that you are well hydrated, and also keep some water with you which you may need during the class. Pilates is by no means aerobic in its execution, but it does use an incredible amout of energy.

Chapter 8 :
Pilates Mat Exercises – Warming Up

Your first Pilates Mat Exercises

Before you begin your mat exercises, your instructor will take you through the way that you should breath when you are in the class. Unlike many other exercise routines, the breathing in Pilates is decidedly slower, and are counted in 4 breaths. Your instructor will usually request that you take slow inhalations that are quite deep through your nose, though in some cases, you will be asked to vary your breathing between your nose and your mouth.

If you have done yoga before, you will be familiar with breathing that goes through your abdomen. With Pilates, your breathing is not centered on your abdomen and instead, you focus your breathing on filling up your lungs. This means that your abdomen does not get raised as you do the mat exercisees, allowing you to keep your abdomen muscles tight dueing your workout.

Here are your first mat exercises. These are designed to help you develop your core strength, as well as establish some stability and increase the flexibility of your body.

Warming Up

You will begin your Pilates session by warming your body up so that you can execute the mat exercises to perfection. This is because they offer te fundamental Pilaets movements, and ensure that you remains as safe as possible when executing the movements.

Begin with breathing by doing the Ron's Clock exercise. You will stand up straight and tall, and maintain a good postude. Ensure that you spine has been lenghtened and that you arms are rounded down by your sides. Your arms should resemble the relaxed stance of a ballerina. Next, inhale through your nose and ensure that you laterally expend your ribs. Then exhale through the mouth and focus on the closure of your ribs. Your arms should be a reflection of the way that your ribs are moving.

Now inhale twice through your nose and expand the ribs. Your arms should be raise a little as you do this. Then you will exhale twice through your mouth, and as you do so, lower your arms this closing your ribs. The difference in this part of the exercise is the increased level that your arms will reach.

Continue with thie exercise, by inhaling and exhaling three times, then four times and so on until you reach six times. With each inhale, your arms should be raised slighlty higher and higher. By the time you reach the 6th inhalation, your arms will be at the 3.00 o'clock position.

If you want a real challene, keep at this breathing exercise until you can put your arms up the the 12 o'clock position.

Imprinting

The next warm up exercise that you should try is known as imprinting. With the exercise, you will lie down gflat on your back and have your arms out by your sides. Then bend your knees and ensure that you keep your feet down flat on the floor. Also, do not worry about the positioning of the spine. It can rest in its natural curves.

This requires you to relax all of your muscles systematically. You will begin by relaxing your shoulders by allowing them to release out on to the floor. Once these are relaxed, move towards your rib cage, allowing this to rest on the floor. Your jaw and throat follow as you release any tension you are holding in this area. Follow with your abdominal muscles which should feel as though they are dropping down towards your spines. With your spine, allow yourself to melt into the floow. Finally, keep your knees and legs in alignment, but relax your hips and your legs as well.

The next thing that you need to do is visualise. Picutre your spine lengthening and then sinking into the mat and once it does this, it should leave a light imprint on the mat. As you are visualising this, you need to relax and monitor your breathing. Your breathing should be deep and fill up your lungs with each inhale.

Picture yourself getting up and as you do so, you are leaving an imprint behind you that reveals your body is perfectly balanced. This warm up exercise should take you approximtely 5 minutes from start to finish.

Pelvic Curl

This is a warm up exercise that will prepare your abdominal muscles and your spine for the Pilates workout. The purpose of this warm up is to assist in the coordination of breath and movement.

To begin with, you need to lie down on your back. Ensure that your knees are bent and that your feet are down flat on the floor. Your geet, ankles and knees should be aligned, and held at a hip distance apart. As you ensure that they are aligned, the natural curves of your spine will be in place.

Next, inhale deeply allowing your breath to go through your chest, move on to your belly and all the way down to the perlvic floor. And then exhale. Release the breath starting from the pelvic floor, moving through the belly and coming out at the chest. Inhale.

Now, as you exhale, you need to carry out a pelvic lift. This means that you engage the muscles in your abdomen and then pull your belly button down. Your abs should do the work of pressing your lower spine down into the floor. The position will have your pubic bone being higher up than your hip bones.

With the next inhale, press down through your feet, which will result in your tail bone starting to curl upwards towards the ceiling. Your hips should be raised, followed by the lower spine and moving up to the middle spine. Your legs need to remain parallel.

Now exhale, and slowly start moving your spine so that it ends up completely settling on the floor. You should feel as though you are going through this process vertebrae by vertabrae, and then stop your exhale once your spine has settled compeltely on the floor.

You should end up back in the natural spine position. Repeat this process a maximum of 5 times to warm up.

Arm Reach and Arm Pull

This is an warm up exercise that you will find yourself coming back to regularly during your Pilates workout. It requires you to warm up your shoulder blades, helping you learn how to find a stable position for them as you exercise.

To start with you need to stand up straight, ensuring that you keep your weight balanced ovver your feet. The top of your head should feel as though you are reaching for the sky, and your shoulders should be as relaxed as possible.

Next, place your arms to your sides so that you are standing in a perfectly straight line. Imagine the way a soilder would take his stance, although yours should not be as rigid.

Now you need to bring your arms up so that they are parallel to the floor. They should extend sraigh out from your shoulders, and your shoulders should not be raised as you extend them. Your shoulders should feel as though they are sliding down your back and your posture should remain unaffected by your moving arms.

Swan Prep

This is a warm up exercise that works to extend your entire body and you will also refer to it often as a counter stretch when you are executing your mat exercises during a Pilates workout.

It is an exercise which will expand the chest, and at the same time, stretch out the abdominals and the quadriceps.

To being this exercise, lie down on the mat with your face down and ensure taht you arms have been kept close tyo your bpdy. Then begin to bend your elbows and while you ar doind so, bring your hands in under your shoulders. Your legs should be kept together.

Using your abdominal muscles, life your belly button up and away from the mat. You will hold a position where your abdominals remain lifted through the entire exercise.

Now, inhale. As you do so, you will lengthen your spine, and this is meant to help send energy all the way from the top of your head towards your upper body to offer support. While you are in this position, your elbows will remain close to your body, your head is meant to stay in line with your spin and your hips should remain firmly on the mat.

Next, exhale and while you do so, ensure that your abdominals are lifted as you release the arc. You will then lengthen your spins as your torso begins to slowly return to the mat sequentially. You should feel as though you are bringing down your lower belly, your mid belly, your lower ribs and so on until you are lying down again.

This warm up exercise should be done at least five times.

Wall Roll Down

This is an excellent warm up exercise if you need to learn how you can better utilise your abdominal muescle, especially when you want to master how to do an articulated curvature of the spine. This type of curvature is the basis of many excercises in Pilates, and being able to master it makes it easier to advance to more complicated levels of Pilates.

To begin with this warm-up, you should stand up tall against a wall. Make sure that your body is 'stuck'to the wall, and then using your feet, walk forward about six inches from the wall.

Make sure that you pull in your abdominal muscles tight as you do this, and ensure that your shoulders are upright. Your chest should also be spread otu wide, and your ribs should be in the down position. Now, raise up your arms, and put them above your head. Hold them up as straight as possible.

Now you will use your neck to being the curve. Keeping your arms up, begin to nod your head and as you do so, your spine will slowly being to roll down and away from the wall. Picture your back doing this bone by bone.

The further you roll yourself forward the deeper you should scoop your abs. Do this in a slow and gently manner. In the way that you were stuck to the wall, picture yourself peeling your way off that wall. Keep you head and neck fully relaxed throughout this process.

When you have gone as low as you can go, your back should be off the wall, but your hips should still be stuck to it. You should be unable to suck your abdominal muscles in any further. You will also begin to feel your hamstrings getting stretched out.

The final part of this arm up is moving back into the original position. This will take some intense working of your abdominal muscles. Begin to work your way back yp the wall, by using your lower abdominal muscles to push you forward. Just as you peeled yourself off the wall bone by bone, send yourself back up in the same way.

Once your back is fully on the wall, you should be back in the upright position, with your hands overhead and your full body stretched out and relaxed.

When preparing your warm ups, you need to choose at least two to three exercises, and aim to complete the warm up session within twenty minutes. There warm ups are ideal for getting ready for some intense mat workouts, which will develop your core strength.

Chapter 9 :
Pilates Mat Exercises – Your Abdominals

Now that you are all warmed up, you can begin some Pilates mat exercises. The next few chapters shall take you through seven exercises that you should attempt, and once you complete these exercises, you are guaranteed to have give your body an exellent workout.

To begin with are three exercises that will help to build your abdominals.

Chest Lift

This is a mat exercise that will help you to develop your upper abs. Although it resembles a crunch, it is very different from one. To execute this mat exercise, you should follow these steps.

1. Begin by lying down on your back on the mat. Your knees need to be bent and your feet should be down flat on the flooor. Your legs should also be parallel. If one was to view the position that you are in, you should appear to be in a straight line with your hips, knees and ankles all in alignment. The toes should be pointing directly away from you.

   In this position, you will be lying down on your spine. For now, ensure that you maintain a natural curve to your spine, which will give you a little lift off the mat.

2. Ensure that your shoulders are down on the mat. Then, bring up your hands and place them behind your head,

allowing your finger tips to touch. You will find that it is your hands which are supporting the back of your skull, and then keep your elbows open. At this juncture, your position will resemble what you would be doing if carrying out abdominal curls.

3. While you are in this position, breath in deeply. As you breathm observe the balance of your body. Make sure that your neck is relaxed and you should feel as though your ribs are dropped. This will be similar to the imprinting that you practiced when you were warming up.

4. Now exhale out, and while doing so, you should pull your belly button down towards your spine. The more you do this, the more your spine will lengthen and this will ensure that your lower back comes down onto the mat. While this is happening, you should tilt your chin a little bit dowen from the top of your head, and with an extended neck, slowly begin to lify your upper spine off your mat. You should stop when the base of your shoulder blades is on the mat. You will feel as though your bottom ribs are going deeper into you as you do this.

5. Pause for a moment, and then draw your abdominals in deeper with an inhale.

6. Exhale, and as you do so, ensure that you keep your abdominals drawn in.

7. At this inhale, return your back to its natural position. You can repeat this a total of 8 times.

Perfecting this move is crucial if you want to move to the next level of difficulty in Pilates. This is the move that will help you accomplish other positions, including the hundred and the single leg stretch.

The Hundred

This is a mat exercise that goes up one level of difficulty from the chest life. It is ideal for beginners to Pilates who have had a little practice and managed to perfect some of the most basic warm up exercises. It also works on the abdominal muscles, and will offer good breathing technique practice.

Whenever you start a Pilates class, this exercise is often done as it allows your body to really warm up the lungs and the abdominals. Coordination is key, as is excellent and strong movement. The more you progress, the more you will modify this exercise in different ways to suit your workouts.

Below are the steps that you need to follow to execute the hundred.

1. Begin by lying down on your back. Whereas in most Pilates exercises you are supposed to allow for the natural curvature of your back, this one is a little different. In this exercises, you will have your knees bend in the tabletop position, where your shins and your ankles will lie parallel to the floor. Once you are in this position, take a deep inhale.

   (The table top position requires you to lie on your back and have your knees bent with your feet off the ground. Your thighs will then be perpendicular to the floor. It is a transitional position allowing you to change positions or begin your workouts with ease)

2. Now you can exhale. As you let the air out of your lungs, bring your head up and keep your chin down. You will make use of your abdominal muscles, and then curve your upper spine so that it is off the floor. This lift will go all the way up to the base of your shoulder blades. Your abdominal muscles should be taut at this point, and will remain that way until the end of your exercise. You need to ensure that your shoulders are engaged at the back. If you are to follow you gaze, you would find yourself looking into the scoop of your abs. Hold this position until you complete a slow exhale, and then inhale again.

3. As you exhale, ensure that you tighten your abs and extend out your legs and arms. Your legs need to strectch out towards the wall and the ceiling are in your line of sight. Depending on your level of comfort and skill, you can adjust your legs so that they are up higher. Your legs should be held in posititon as low as possible without you shaking and without your lower spine being pulled off the mat. In the meantime, your arms ahsould extend out straight out, and you should hold them up low just a few inches above the floor with your fingers outstretched.

4. Hold this position, and focus on your breathing. You will need to take in five short breaths, and then breath out five short breaths. As you are doing this breathing, your arms should correspond with some basic pumping. Your abdomnal muscles should be offering you all the support. While doing this exercise, your neck and your shoulders needs to be relaxed

5. The cycle that you have completed in point four should be repeated until you have completed a cycle of ten full

breaths. This means that you will complete a total of ten cycles of the five short breaths in and the five short breaths out, remembering that you need to keep yoru arms pumping. For support, your back will be flat on your spine.

6. Now you can finish the exercise. You will need to keep your spine curved and bring your knees up to your chest. Hold on yo your knees and ensure that your upper spine rools down gently until you have your head back down to the floor. Inhale and exhale.

Rolling Like A Ball

This is the third abdominal exercise that you should master, as it is used in all Pilates mat exercises. Developing your skill in this exercise is an excellent way to stimulate your spine as well as build on your abdominals.

To get into this exercise, you should follow these steps.

1. Start out by sitting down on your mat as if in a lotus position with your legs crossed. Then, clasp your hands over your shins, holding the position above your ankles.

2. Next, you wioll be makring a curve in your back. To do this, you need to drop your shoulders down and use this movement to widen your back. Tighten your abdominal muscles and ensure that your neck is part of the curve that has appeared. In this position, you should avoid tucking in your head as this interferes with the curve.

3. Now, you should life your feet off the mat and place most of your weight on to your bottom. Use these muscles to hold you balance.

4. While in this position inhale, and suck in your lower abs. Then you should roll your abdominal to roll back up until your shoulders. It should feel like a fluid movement. Then you should pause for a moment.

5. Now you can exhale. As you do so, keep your spine curved in a deep scoop. Using your abdominal muscles, make sure that you return to an upright position. It is necessary to hold your balance. Repeat this exercises 6 times.

If you find that your position does not exactly resemble a curve, you should take note of what you are doing with your abs. If your abs are appropriately taught, then you will make a curve with no problem.

These are three exercises that build up your abdominals. Now for some more exercise that focus on other parts of your body.

Chapter 10 :
Pilates Mat Exercises – Your Legs

This chapter feature three exercises that you can do to build on your legs using Pilates. Once you complete it, you will have given your legs a complete workout, strenthening them and building up on their overall flexibility. These exercises are also meant to build up on your core strength, becase as much as they are focused on your legs, they will also work on your abdominals and shoulders. If you are looking to tone and strengthen, these are ideal.

One Leg Circle

The first mat exercise for your legs that you will work on is the one leg circle. This exercise needs a good amount of concentration, as your will need to control your movements, be precise and breath well for it to be effective. It is appropriate for a beginner and once mastered, can be incorporated into any Pilates workout that you execute. Here are the steps that you need to follow.

1. Get into the right position by lying down on your back, ensuring that your legs are extended out before you on the floor. Leep your arms by your sides and practice imprinting for a moment. While doing this, you should ensure that your weight feels balanced, particularly on your hips and your shoulders. Inhale deeply and exhale several times until you feel as though your body is fully relaxed.

2. Your then need to bring your abdominals into the forefront of this exercise by pulling them taught and keeping them help in. This will ensure that your pelvis

is anchored and your shoulders are held in place. Now that you are in this firm position, extend one of your legs upwards, making sure that your toes are pointing towards the ceilings. Make sure that you feel the stretch in your hamstrings, and that you keep your hips flat as you extend your stretch. If it feels like there is too much strain on your hamstrings, bend your knees slightly.

3. Now, you are ready to do some leg circles. As you inhale use your extended leg and cross it towards the opposite hip. Try and keep your knees as straight as possible, and have your hips in place. Then exhale, and drop the leg down a little. Using control, take your straight led and sweep it around in a small circle. You should end up back in yoru starting position. The only part of your body that should be moving is your leg.

4. Repeat this motion with five circles. Once you have completed these, switch legs. Complete two sets of this exercise.

Saw

This is a leg exercise that is designed to work on your back and hamstrings. It will stretch the, well and also offer some work to your pelvis. This exercise requires some preparation before you can go fully into it and you can complete the exercise following three simple phases. Here are details on the phases that you will follow.

1. **Phase one** – Begin by sitting upright on your mat, ensuring that most of your weight is being pushed down into your bottom. You should visualize that the weight is moving all the way from the top of your head and then resting at your bottom from here. Make sure that

43

your legs are extended forward in front of you. Rather than keeping them together, have them positioned at a shoulder width apart. You may need to use a prop like a rolled towel under your hips if you feel that your hamstrings are way too tight. Stretch out your arms to the side and hold this position.

2. **Phase two** – Take in a deep breath. As you do so, begin to twist your entire torso so that your left arm is reaching out to your right foot. Use your abdominal muscles to keep yourself grounded as the only parts of you that should be moving are your arms and your torso. As you exhale, you should turn your upper torso so that is appears as though you are about to curl into yourself. Your abdominal muscles will keep you grounded. Exhale and repeat this with the other hand and leg. You can repeat this several times, extended your arms a little more each time.

3. **Phase three** – Once you have reached the furthest point of your stretch, take in a deep inhale and slowly return to your sitting position. As you exhale, move your body until you are back to your starting position. Your hamstrings should be filling quite warm by the end of this exercise.

Side Kick

These are leg exercises which are meant to tone and strengthen the hips as well as the thigs and the abs. They work by using your core muscles to stabilise your upper body, meaning that your lower body is able to move independently. Here is how you can begin these exercises.

1. Start be lying down on your mat on your side. Ensure that you have lined up your ears with your shoulders, hips, knees and ankles.

2. Use your arm to prop up your head, and while you do so, make sure that your back and neck do not go out of alighment.

3. Take your other hand and use it to press down onto the mat in the front of your chest. Your hand should be placed with the palm down. Your stability will not come from the positioning of your arm, rather, it should come from your abdominal muscles. Therefore, the arm does not need to offer you any balance.

4. Now, move your legs forward so that they are a little infront of the hips. Then from the hips, rotate them in a slow motion. Before you move further, check on your line up. Your entire body should still be alinged, though your knees and your ankles will now be infront of you.

Now that you are in position, there is a series of kicks that you can attempt that will work with your entire lowe body. These include: -

- The Kick Front – With this kick, you need to lift up your leg several inches. Flexing the muscles, visualise bursts of energy moving into your body from the heel of the foot. Once you have the muscle tightened, make sure that you can swing your top leg to your front.Once you have extended it to the front, do a small pulse kick.

- The Length to the Back – Pointing your toes outwards, take the top led and sweep it to the back and hold this poistion. After a few seconds, flex all the muscles in your leg by tightening them. Then kick to the front and loosen the muscles.

- The Kick Up – Make sure that your body is properly aligned and that your shoulders and your upper torso is being kept firmly in place. Remember to keep your abdominal muscles pulled in. Lengthen your leg and then kick it up towards the ceiling.

- The Inner Thigh Lift – This is a different type of kick that will work on your inner thighs. Your starting position will remain the same except for your top arm and leg which will see a difference in the position that is adopted. To begin with, nring the foot of your top leg upwards and allow if to find a postion in the front of your hips. Then using your top hand, take a hold of the ouside of your ankle. Once you are in this position, breathe in and keep the bottom leg straight. Use your inner thigh muscles and then raise your leg slightly so that it is ajust a few inches off the floor. As you exhale, keep the length of your legs and then lower it to the ground slowly.

When executing your side kick exercises, you should repeat each of them at least 5 times for the maximum effect.

You should attempt to complete at least 2 different leg exercises at each session that you have Pilates. Try and alternate them regularly so that over a period, you offer your entire leg an excellent workout.

Chapter 11 :
Pilates Mat Exercises – Your Back

The seventh exercise that you can try on a mat is a back exercise. Pilates is excellent for strenghening your back and also for working on your arms and your shoulders. In addition to strenghtening the core, the work that is done on the back will help improve your overall posture by leaps and bounds, increasing the strength that is carried around all through your body. Here is an excellent exercise that you can use for your back.

The Pilates Plank

This exercise will almost always appear in your Pilates session, whether you are a beginner or have acquired some skill. This is because it is ideal for anyone looking to deveop their stability as well as increase on their core strength. It also woks like a regular plank, as it offers benefits that wll be felt in the entire body.

The Pilates plank in many ways resembles what you can expect to see in a refuly push up. The difference is that in this exercise there is minimal strain that is placed on the uipper body and the shoulders and neck particulalry do not experience too much strain.

To do this exercise, you should follow these steps

1. Start by lying face down on your mat. Then get on to your knees. When in this position, place your hands on the floor right in front of your, and ensure that your fingers are positioned to point ahhead. Keep your arms as straight as possible, but do not lock your elbows.

47

2. Then you should tighten your abdominal muscles and once taut, lenghthen your spine. Visualise that there is energy moving through your body and it is starting out at the top of your head, and making its way through your body all the way to your tail bone.

3. Now, lean forward, and ensure that the weight of your body is in your hands. Your shoulders should be aligned over your wrists. If for any reason you begin to feel pain in your wrist due to placing your weight on it, you should lift it up occasionally and this will help to relieve any pressure.

4. Now that you have your arms in position, with your abdominals well held in, begin to extend your legs out so that they are straight behind you. Ensure that you have kept them close together. Visualise the energy in your body soaring through your legs and going directly to your heels.

5. Your toes should be under your feet, ensuring that any weight is being carried by the balls of your feet. Tighten the muscles all through your feet, but ensure that you do not clench down on your bottom muscles.

6. While in this position, hold it and breath in deeply. While you inhale, you should feel some expansion on your lower ribs as well as on your back. Hold this position and continue with slow inhaling and exhaling at least five times before you release it.

When you have completed the plank, you will feel muscles all over your body warm up, and you may also feel a gentle strain on some of them. This exercise is powerful for developing total body strength, and it can be done by even a beginner at Pilates.

Chapter 12:
Comparative analysis- Pilates vs. Yoga

Choosing and diagnosing the right therapy for your body is no less than a challenge. This entails both the physical as well mental therapies. Having so much advancement in every field of medicine as well as the physical sciences, all of us are surrounded by plenty of choices and options. But this excessiveness is also enhancing the confusions as well as misinterpretations. People get whirled by these options because there raises a long held debate on all types of options and alternatives. Every single method has millions of followers along with same number of opponents, who are making the debates more long and complicate. Many groups fallaciously deem that Pilates is like other forms of exercises, only with a changed name. But whatever form of exercise you are using you should have an in depth understanding regarding the purpose, possible alternatives and the core theme for each type of exercise. The major form of exercise with which Pilates is mostly mixed or assorted, is Yoga. One cannot affirm or rule out that Pilates scheme is more effective than Yoga or vice versa but the underlying basics is that one should know how to differentiate between the two and how to choose the method appropriate for the particular needed of the body.

Pilates vs. Yoga

- Picking and deciding between these two techniques is quite crucial and critical because it demands for a systematic analysis and thoughtful reasoning.

- For the supporters of yoga or Pilates, their particular situate of calisthenics is the best preference presented. And they are rather defensible in the sense that they choose the respective set if exercise for attainment of their particular goals and agendas.

- As far as Yoga is concerned the core of this scheme is focus on breathing so that the human movements and functions get tuned with the rhythm and harmony of breathing patterns. Moreover the technique is also considered as a technique of soul. Yogis usually connote that the human soul and body must be moving and struggling in one single direction.

- On the other hand Pilates is a scheme with the central attention towards body movements and postures. Although breathing is a major section for the hub of Pilates, practitioner, yet it entails supremacy to be related with central muscles of human body.

- As far as the historical perspectives are concerned, Pilates can be regarded as a set of contemporary techniques, developed in the modern era of progress and development. Whereas Yoga connotes a technique which has a long reported history of even two or more centuries back. so as far as the alterations is concerned Pilates has been subjected t little alterations as compared to Yoga, which after passing from generation to generation has merged with a number of different cultural aspects and demographic inclinations.

- As largely followed rule of thumb if the goal is to get solid muscular abdominal region than people chose Pilates as the most appropriate way, but for concentration and focus achievements, Yoga is the largely focused technique.

- Pilates is based on a number of finely tuned apparatus and movement machines for delivering the accurate and required results according to the customized and desired goals of very individual. Whereas Yoga can be practiced without any automation kit, definite breathing designs are involved and focused in yoga.

Chapter 13:
Precautionary Measures and Concluding Remarks

A major contribution and consequence of Pilates is the intense help in gaining the eventual control and charge of the body so that nothing can affect the human body. But any people believe that Pilates is not effective only because they had been unable to get to the real way of practicing and extracting the techniques of Pilates. But on the other side of the picture, Pilates has emerged as a revolutionary aid for many others who have lived upon this technique for years and years. The distinctive method is a diverse set of ideas governing and maintaining human body and soul in an unparallel way.

Some may label it unsuccessful because their mind has a permanent impression of fruitless exercises because of some previous bad experience. Again the root cause lies in implementing the method accurately. Pilates also affects the brain parts, many people have reported that the activity of brain cells is largely triggered by this distinguishing method of body flow and movement, so that one is able to get an eventual control and concern towards all the functions of human body and mind.

In the end we will suggest all those who have looked upon this book that they should start focusing on their strengths and weaknesses. Physical health is not something which can be put down in ignore list, rather it should be in the priority list so that one s able to extract the maximum benefit out of this world and its blessings.

Pilates is no doubt a challenging technique if you want to get full benefits of it with long-lasting and wider benefits. But once you get on the track nothing is impossible. Start working on extracting the methods of getting mastery over this technique. Some initial faults in your method of implementation may not be the indicators of failure of this method. It is not also a hit and trial method in which you can make deletions and additions with your own prescriptions. It is a long held rule of exercise and physical output that needs to be implemented in its true spirits.

The attainment and gratification of physical rigor, mental tranquil and divine serenity is incalculably precious to their individuals if someone gets this miraculous combination, in today's world of fuss and messed up routines. However, it is not the matter of gaining these blessings; the real task is to maintain this exclusive combination of effectiveness from human body to human soul and subconscious. One simple way is to start practicing Pilates from today and the eventual results will be overwhelming for all of us, in terms of healthier and more effective societies. Together we can bring the cumulative development and vitality.

Although you have all this information on Pilates at your fingertips, there are possibly some questions that you may have about this type of exercise, and this section explains why Pilates is right for you.

Easy to learn

Despite what many may believe, Pilates is easy to learn and master, and with time and practice, can be done anywhere that is convenient for you. The aspects that make it easy to learn are the fact that there is no need for one to have strength to begin. By practicing Pilates, you will build up your strength. In addition, you do not need to have any coordination. The exercises are designed to develop your coordination. In addition, one should not be concerned about flexibility. Unlike similar exercises, with Pilates, there is minimal contortion into different shapes. Instead it is all about easy stretches. Experience is also unnecessary as you can begin from scratch no matter what your level of fitness, and build yourself up.

To get the most out of your Pilates sessions, you should be prepared and motivated to give in your very best effort. Even the exercises that seem a little challenging can be quickly mastered if you have the motivation to see them through. The moment that you feel uncomfortable or under strain, stop the exercise. You will not lose anything by doing so, and you can choose to try something else that will be of better comfort for you.

No Pain, No Gain

The heading of this point is a term that you probably associate with most exercise regimes, but it does not apply when you are doing Pilates. Following your classes, you will likely experience some soreness, but this is far from being described as painful. It also depends on how fit you were before you started the Pilates classes. If you were at a very low level of fitness, you will likely feel much sorer than if you have been actively exercising in the past.

Safe Results

Pilates is excellent for people of all ages, whether your or old because it is safe to try out. In addition, it offers effective exercises, helping to tone and strengthen the entire body, while also helping one to lose weight if they need to. There are a range of ailments that can be improved once you start to practice Pilates. If you are having problems with your balance,

Pilates can help with that. The same applies to improvement of your posture substantially.

Pilates can be skewed towards meeting your specific health and lifestyle needs. Therefore, if you are a pregnant woman, overweight, totally inflexible, an athlete, or even recovering from some sort of body or muscular injury, you can still find some Pilates exercises that will be safe for you to practice.

Chapter 14 :
Commonly Used Pilates Terms

With your knowledge of Pilates from this book, you are now ready to attempt some Pilates at home, or to join a beginners Pilates class. Whether you choose to use some videos to help you work out, or you prefer to be with an instructor, there are some terms that you will hear which you need to be familiar with. This final chapter explains those terms to you, and will help you to be in the know when you are enjoying your Pilates experience.

Here are the terms in alphabetic order for your ease of reference.

- **Abdominals** – These are the muscles that you will find at the front of your torso. They include several muscle groups and are also known as the core muscles. These muscle groups are the rectus abdominis, transversus abdominis and internal obliques. In short, they are also referred to as abs, abdominal muscles and stomach muscles.

- **Abductor** – There refer to a group of muscles which will take a particular body part a distance away from the midline of the body. When you are in class and doing side leg kick ups, you are likely to hear this term.

- **Core Strength** – This refers to the balanced development of your muscles. Specifically, the muscles in question are those that offer your entire body some stability, adn that you use when creating alighnment. These are the muscles which you will use when you want to move the trunk of your body. They include your abdominals and the muscles on your back.

- **Counter Stretch** – This looks at changing the direction with which you stretch your body. What it requires is for you to stretch your body in the opposite direction from an exercise that you have just completed. The aim of this is to streth the muscles that may be opposing.

- **Eccentric Contraction** – When you add the element of force to a Pilates exercise, you are likely to hear this term. It is when you lengthen the muscle as it is contraction due to resisting some sort of force.This is most often done when you are executing leg exercises.

- **Flexion** – This is a term that refers to the flexing of your muscles. When you flex your muscles you are decreasing the angle of the muscles between certain parts. What usually happens is that you bring certain parts of your body closer together as a result of flexing.

- **Neurtal Spin** – When you are doing any exercise, there is a way that your spine will take shape when you lie down. Most times, people will tense up their spines. In Pilated, it is necessary to start some positions with a neutral spine. This is basically the natural way that you would position your spine once you have allligned all of your body parts well. This means that in this position, you would be following the natural curves of your back, rather than trying to flatten your back out.

- **Oppositional Stretch** – This term defines a stretch that when carried out is able to extend the body in two different directions at the same time. This is often found when you need to do some leg exercies, and you may need to point your head in another direction.

- **Scoop the Abs** – This is a term that you will hear when your instructor wants you to tighten up your abdominal muscles and pul them in towards your spine. You should appear to be leaving an expanse in the abdominal area.

- **Sit Bones** – These are those parts of your bottom that feel bony when you are sitting upright on a surface that is firm.

Conclusion

Pilates is an excellent way for you to bring your body life, and it also has the added advantage of stimulating your mind. When you begin to put these exercises into practice, you will find that in a short while, your entire body will begin to function better from the inside out.

That is because Pilates is an exercise system that is designed to change your being in a positive way. What is great about this system is that it has no restrictions. Any person can try it, and will see positive results from doing so. If you are at a low level of fitness, you will find that the exercises are simple and you can execute them without experiencing pain, or strain.

Now that you have a detailed list of the exercises that you can practice, it is time that you took matters into your own hands and began your journey into Pilates. Use the information in this book to familiarize yourself with the techniques, and if you are able to, add in the support of a trained and certified Pilates professional.

This book touches on what you need to conquer the basics of Pilates. The more you practice, the easier it will be for you to increase your level of difficulty and transition into using more complicated apparatus and additional instruments for practice.

I hope this book was able to help you to start living your life as you should. The next step is to apply what you've learned on a daily basis. Take the opportunity now to transform your entire body. There are few body movement exercises that have such a profound effect on you from the inside out. By making Pilates a part of your every day existence, you are welcoming a bright and fulfilling future with open arms.

Yoga

The Ultimate Guide for Beginners

How to Practice Yoga and Have Happiness, Balance and Strength Back to Your Life

Table of Contents

Chapter 1:
Introduction

This book contains proven steps and strategies on how to get started with the practice of yoga and take advantage of the numerous benefits it can offer. It features comprehensive information on yoga and its numerous benefits. Also included in this book are practical tips on how to get started with the practice of yoga, some diet tips as well as some yoga etiquette to bear in mind when practicing yoga.

Yoga is defined as an organized practice of exercise, meditation, positive thinking, diet control, relaxation and breath which is aimed at producing harmony in the environment, mind and body. The practice of yoga involves low-impact physical movements, meditation, relaxation, breathing strategies (called Pranayama) and poses (called Asanas). A lot of people are familiar with yoga positions although most are not aware that the practice of yoga involves much more.

In the field of medicine, yoga strategies are being employed for the promotion of overall health, in substance abuse treatment strategies as well as complementary treatment strategy for illnesses such as HIV/AIDS, cancers, coronary heart problems, depression and anxiety disorders. The practice of yoga is considered as a low-cost self-help strategy to overall wellness.

The word yoga is derived from the Sanskrit term "Yog", which means union. Yoga is described then as a union of the bodily systems with the mind's consciousness. In philosophy, yoga creates a union of energy (spirit or soul), mind and body to produce a state of calmness or equanimity. Advancing more, combining philosophy and science, an individual will experience the union of internal energy, mind, body and cosmic forces leading to better physical, mental health and finally self-realization.

Some history of Yoga

The roots of yoga are rooted during the ancient times in India. Yoga is a traditional system of mental and physical practices that originated in South Asia during the Indus Valley civilization. The basic objective of yoga is to promote harmony in the mind, body and the environment.

Yoga involves a holistic system of social, mental, spiritual and physical development. For over a thousand of years, the philosophies of yoga was passed on from the master teacher to its students, it was around 200 BC when the very first written records of the practice of yoga first appeared in Yogasutra of Patanjali. The system of yoga includes the Asthangayoga or the eightfold path.

In Western countries, a number of yoga schools are popular and employs some or all the limbs of Asthangayoga as described by Patanjali. Following are the eight limbs:

1. Samadhi – ultimate superior meditation strategies and psychic methods achieved after the regular practice for general consciousness

2. Dhyana – concentration strategies for mental calmness and balance

3. Dhana – concentration strategies for mental calmness and balance

4. Pratihara – strategies for separating the mind from the other senses to achieve mental calmness and balance

5. Pranayama – breathing strategies for mental and physical balance

6. Asaana – posture strategies for mental and physical balance this is what a lot of people perceive as yoga.

7. Niyama – strategies for purifying and managing self

8. Yama – rules for effective and successful living in community

Chapter 2:
The Benefits of Yoga

The numerous beneficial effects of different yoga techniques include improved body flexibility, stress reduction, boosted performance and achievement of inner peace and self-realization. The yoga techniques has been promoted as complementary treatment strategy to help in the treatment or various diseases such as asthma, anxiety disorders, depression, coronary heart problems as well as extensive rehabilitation for illnesses such as traumatic brain injury and musculoskeletal problems. The techniques of yoga have also been recommended as behavioral treatment for substance abuse (such as alcohol and drug abuse) and smoking cessation.

If you attend yoga classes, you may take advantage of the following benefits:

1. Spiritual

   - Contentment

   - Tranquility and inner peace

   - Life with direction, purpose and meaning

2. Mental

   - Intellectual enhancement, which leads to and enhanced decision-making skills

   - Relief and prevention from stress-associated disorders

- Relief of stress brought about by successful emotional control

3. Physical

- Improved immune system

- Increased energy levels

- Weight control

- Relaxation of muscular strength

- Improved abdominal strength

- Improved digestion

- Improved cardiovascular endurance

- Improved balance and body flexibility

At this point, a word of caution with regard to the inappropriate practice of yoga is necessary. With the endless advantages may come injury for beginners or those individuals who practice it without adequate instructions. More than 18 million Americans around the world are reported to employ some form of yoga and medical experts as well as health care providers are recording injuries such as cartilage tears; back and neck pains; and ligament and muscle sprains.

Yoga societies recommend at least 100 hours of training under the supervision of a yoga experts. About 5,000 yoga instructors all over the world reportedly have satisfied that requirement. Before attending a particular yoga class, inquire about the training and credentials of the yoga instructor.

Before committing yourself to a set program, you may wish to sit on a class and observe first.

- **Yoga for Specific Health Problems**

- Multiple sclerosis – According to experts from the Oregon Health and Science University, some type of yoga forms may help lessen fatigue in individuals suffering from multiple sclerosis (MS). These experts have employed the Iyengar form of yoga for individuals suffering from MS.

- Rheumatoid Arthritis – 1.3 million of Americans are reported to be suffering from rheumatoid arthritis. 75 percent of this population is women. Yoga may be beneficial for people suffering from arthritis for pain and stiffness relief, improvement of the range of motion and boost strength for everyday activities.

- Individuals who are elderly or inactive – if you love a sedentary lifestyle, yoga may be the most suitable exercise for both the body and mind to start your active life. Yoga also helps to lessen stress in addition to improving the posture and strengthening the muscles and bones. Since you really do not have to be at the optimum physical shape in order to do yoga, it is the most ideal activity for inactive people as well as for the elderly who might not otherwise engage in exercise.

Ongoing Research on the Benefits of Yoga

The National Institutes of Health is currently assessing yoga as an alternative treatment for insomnia, chronic lower back pain and other disorders.

Chapter 3:
Yoga Etiquette that You Need to Know

Good manners may seem really hard to come by especially in our over-worked, stressed out community. We may all use some yoga now more than ever. Along with its promise for a healthier well-being and deep inner peace, it is no surprise that the ancient practice of yoga continues to be very popular in the Western countries. A recent yoga journal reported that about 14 million individuals in the United States alone have practiced some form of yoga in 2010. With the ever growing of yogis, occasional ruffled feathers may tend to be unavoidable. Below are some yoga etiquettes to observe when attending yoga classes:

1. Be quiet please. This may seem like a no-brainer. Before attending a yoga class, make sure to turn off your cell phone. It will also be a very bad idea to make a loud entrance or exit in yoga class. Just a little reminder just like in the movie theater before the show starts, please be quiet or make as little noise as possible while you get settled for your yoga class.

2. If you show up late, tiptoe in class

    Showing up late in yoga class in very inevitable, but it would be very polite to wait until everybody is finished with their starting meditation and be as quiet as a mice as not to interrupt with the peace.

3. During the Dharma talk, be respectful by making eye contact with your yoga instructor

    Eye contact is very much a strong manifestation of respect. When your instructor is talking about how the practice of yoga have modified their life or sharing certain traditional philosophy teachings; give your undivided, full attention. Even if you do not like the manner your instructor is providing the material, try your very best to keep concentrated. So instead of closing your eyes or lying down, be attentive. You may just discover something new from your yoga instructor.

4. Follow what your instructor is teaching and don't try adding your own "flair"

It is very disrespectful when you try to do your own thing. Your yoga instructor places a great deal of effort and time to prepare for the class and do it with great purpose. Your yoga instructor may most likely attended several workshops, read books on yoga and practice regularly to perfect their craft. There is something great about letting yourself to be led and just experience what your instructor has to offer. If there is certain yoga pose that you feel you can't live without, you are always free to do it when your yoga class is over.

5. Attending a yoga class is a "work-in" and not a "workout"

Whenever you take a group exercise session, bike, run or lift weights, you work up a sweat and experience a good workout. Yoga on the other hand, is a traditional system for overall well-being where participants learn to widen the conscious mind deeper into the subconscious mind. The ultimate goal is to learn to live in union with other people and with nature. The principle of yoga is a shift to the inner-most self and a technique to see the divine and true nature. Therefore, it is best to regard yoga as a "work in".

6. Don't take over the skylight

Perhaps you have your favorite spot in the yoga studio – by the windy window, beneath the skylight and right in front of the yoga instructor, however be adaptable. A morning yoga class on a Saturday may get quite jam packed, and you do not wish to be that person who refuses to move his/her mat a few inches to the right since it will ruin the view.

7. Do not walk across other yogis' mats

To look for a spot to roll you matt out, keep from touching other's mat. No one likes another person's sweaty feet to be touching their stuff.

8. Do not laugh

Don't laugh at the old man wearing an American flag in the front row, your friend or even at yourself. However, you should feel free to smile every now and then. Yogis should also know how to have fun.

9. Do not be a human sprinkler

Yoga practice can really get you sweaty, so take a towel with you during every class. Dripping sweat all over the other person's mat next to you is sort of like peeing on another person's carpet. Angry glares are absolutely to take place.

10. Do not rush out of class

If you rush out of class, you may step on innocent hands or knock over water bottles during savasana. Relax, you just spent all that time doing all that yoga poses.

Chapter 4:
Food and Yoga

Diet and food play a crucial role in yoga. The impacts of poor nutrition and inappropriate nutrition uncover themselves in unpleasant appearance and in flawed behavior and thinking. According to the principles of yoga, food is categorized as Rajasic, Tamasic and Sattvic, which is the ancient adaptation of the Good, the Bad and the Ugly.

- Sattvic Yoga Foods

  These are food items which are prepared fresh with limited seasonings or spices. These foods maintain their nutritional value since they are cooked very simply. One of the most delicious and nutritious foods with great benefit on the overall body health is Sprout. The principles of yoga highly recommend Sattvic foods.

- Rajasic Yoga Foods

  These food items are also commonly referred to as foods for kings or of individuals who have energetic or restless dispositions. A huge selection of foods cooked through various methods – fried, baked or highly seasoned, form this yoga food category. Also under this category are processed beverages, alcohol and sweets. By and large, these food items causes additional weight and fats to the body. These foods lead to a feeling of uneasiness after eating and thus produce a lethargic disposition.

- Tamasic Yoga Foods

This category includes non-vegetarian and vegetarian foods which are cooked with hot seasonings, salts and excess spices. As a general perception, these types of foods cause a feeling of laziness to those who eat them. Foods under this category lead to intolerant and rough temperament.

Yoga Diet – Foods to Stay Away From

1. Poor quality oils, margarine and animal fats

2. White flour and white sugar

3. Over-spiced foods

4. Old, stale and over-reheated foods

5. Genetically engineered foods

6. Irradiated and microwaved foods

7. Eggs, fish and meat

8. Fried foods

9. Factory farm dairy products

10. Canned foods (excepts naturally canned tomatoes, vegetables and fruits)

11. Processed, artificial foods

12. Artificial sweeteners

13. Coffee, tea, tobacco, alcohol and all stimulants

Yoga Diet – Foods to Eat

1. Natural sugars such as molasses, maple syrup, honey and jiggery

2. Whole grains such as oats, wheat and rice

3. Lentils and pulses

4. Fresh juices, most especially the lemony kind, natural water and herbal teas

5. Fenugreek, basil, mint, turmeric, coriander, cumin, fennel, cardamom, cinnamon, ginger and other types of sweet spices

6. Slightly salted or roasted nuts such as sesame, pecans, walnuts, coconuts and almonds

7. Dairy products such as cottage cheese, yogurt, ghee and milk from dairy animals which have been well treated

8. Clarified butter (ghee), butter and any other type of natural plant-based oils such as sunflower, olive and sesame

9. Fresh sweet fruits of all sorts, ideally taken whole

10. All types of vegetables, specially green leafy variants

Points to Consider:

How you cook and eat your meals is just as important as what you consume. Cook and consume your food with awareness and love, the same manner that you execute yoga on the mat. Individuals who execute yoga with yoga principles in mind are conscious of this manner of thinking. Cooing or eating your meals while you are distracted, irate or upset can bring about negative impacts such as an upset stomach. Even if you are dining out and the food served to you is not your usual yoga diet standards, blessing the foods and knowingly wanting to take the nourishment and drive out the rest can transform it from a negative to a positive dining experience.

The Key is Moderation

Just as like with any healthy diet, a yoga diet which put emphasis on moderation and balance is the key. This should not only apply to the amount of food but also on the seasonings and other flavorings that are found in it. Excess grease, heavy spices or an overload of spices are not part of a yoga diet, but only fresh pure food items for their nourishment. Overloading your taste buds or your plate places a danger on your mind and disposition.

When Should You Eat

Yoga experts strongly suggest that you must not eat foods 2 to 3 hours prior to a yoga class. Some yogis further recommend that you eat food items that are easy on the digestive system and your stomach. Suggestions include foods like toasted whole-wheat bread, hummus, veggies, rice, low-fat yogurt, apples, pears, oatmeal and bananas. Pre-workout snacks must include foods with low glycemic index and you must avoid simple carbs and sugars such as white bread, sweets and donuts.

Rule Exceptions

Because of health issues, food allergies as well as other factors, a strict yoga diet will not be beneficial for everybody. This is but alright as there are yoga diet variations where yogis can consume meat or fish in order to stay focused and healthy. What's important is that you listen to your body and customize the diet according to your body's needs, rather than sticking to a diet regimen which will only make you feel sick, weary or weak.

Chapter 5:
Yoga Poses for Beginners

So you're about to go to your first yoga class? Then studying these foundation postures should help get you started. These are the very first poses that you will learn as a yoga beginner.

1. Tadasana (Mountain Pose)

    Just because these yoga poses are very simple, doesn't imply that they will be very easy. Placing new awareness to a particular pose you think that you know can actually be very difficult. Mountain pose for example, appears like just plainly standing. However, in the context of yoga, there are really a lot of things going on with this pose:

    - crown of the head rises

    - shoulder blades slide down the back

    - bones are loaded up with the shoulders directly over the hips

    - muscles of the legs are engaged

    - heels root down

    While doing the mountain pose, do not forget to breathe.

2. Urdhva Hastansana (Raised Arms Pose)

    Inhale, then place your arms up over your head. The raised arms pose should be your basic stretch in the morning. Just remember to focus yourself on keeping the proper alignment of the body that you have attained in the mountain pose, specifically keeping it grounded in the heels and maintain your shoulder blades moving away from your ears. You can fix your eyes on your hands as they come up.

3. Uttanasana (Standing Forward Bend)

Exhale then fold your legs over into a forward bend. At first, if the hamstrings feel slightly tight, bend your knees. This will release your spine. Allow your head to hang heavy and slightly straighten your legs if you would like to although keep your head hanging. You may allow your hips to be distance apart or your feet touching, whichever feels better.

4. Malasana (Garland Pose)

Shift your feet out to the mat's edges and bend your knees, going for a squatting pose. If necessary, the toes may turn out. Take a rolled up blanket under them if your heels cannot reach the floor. This is a pose that is very natural for kids however adults lose the knack for it due to age. This pose is good for the hips and to neutralize the adverse impacts of prolonged riding in cars or sitting in chairs. The Garland pose is also a very beneficial yoga pose.

5. The Lunge Position

Straighten up your legs then place your feet back under the hips. Then step your right leg to the back of your yoga mat. For a deeper lunge, bend your left knee. Try placing your bent knee over the ankle to put your left thigh directly parallel to the floor. Keep your right leg strong and straight with your heel reaching back. If this pose is too intense for you, you can alternately drop your right knee to the mat. Before returning the right foot in front of the mat next to the left foot, take five breaths. Do this all over again with the right foot forward and then the left leg back.

6. Plank Position

Following your second lunge pose, place the right foot back so that it will be situated right next to the left foot at the back of your yoga mat. This is the basic groundwork for a push-up. Here, take five breaths while making it sure that your hips do not rise too high or drop too low. If your elbows have a tendency to hyperextend, bend them. Place your knees down if needed. Following the five breaths, place your knees to the mat and return back to sit with your heels. Take a moment to rest.

7. The Staff Position

Allow yourself to catch your breath. Then swing your legs around to allow them to be outstretched in your front. The staff position is actually seated equivalent of the mountain pose. While this also seems like a very simple pose, there are a lot of things going on with this position:

- Arms may be slightly bent or straight

- Shoulders stack over the hips

- Spine straight and long

- Legs stay strong with the feet flexed

8. Paschimottanasa (Seated Forward Bend)

When exhaling, place your torso over your legs in a straight bend. By now, the hamstrings should be warmer than earlier when you were doing the standing forward bend. Keep on breathing, prolonging the spine with every inhale and making your forward fold deeper with every exhale. Keep breathing with the feet flexed.

9. Janu Sirsana (Head to Knee Pose)

Return back up to a sit. Bend your left leg then place the sole of the left sole inside the right thigh. To deepen the position using your breathe; employ the same methods as described above. Following five breaths sit back up and switch legs.

10. Ananda Balasana (Happy Baby Pose)

Lie flat on your back and hug your knees in front of your chest. Then take apart your knees and place every ankle directly over the knee so that the shins are placed perpendicular towards the floor. Then contract your feet and hold on to them from the outer surface as you place your knees downward. If it feels good, roll side to side a little on your sacrum. This is a pose that is well-known to everyone with children. Following five breaths stretch out your legs on the floor. Take a few moments to rest.

11. Balasana (Child's Pose)

The Child's pose is the position that you may assume at any time you feel like taking a break during the yoga session. If you feel overly fatigued or feel light-headed, you do not have to wait for your instructor to call for a break. Feel free to assume the child's pose on your own and return back to class whenever you are ready. It is really up to you, which actually is one the yoga's best learning: stay attuned to the signs that your body is giving you.

12. Chakravakasana (Cat-cow Stretch)

The cat-cow stretch could be the best position that you could learn when beginning to practice yoga, particularly if you are suffering from back pains. Even if you cannot make it to the next yoga session, you may continue doing this pose on your own to promote your spinal health.

13. Adho Mukah Svanasana (Downward Facing Dog)

This pose is almost entirely synonymous with yoga. Starters to yoga usually place themselves too far forward in this pose, making it more like a planking pose, so keep in mind to maintain your weight entirely in your legs, your heels reaching the floor and your butt high. For people with tight hamstrings, this pose may be modified by bending the knees a lot or a little. Eventually the downward facing dog pose becomes a resting position.

Chapter 6:
Yoga Tips for Beginners

To start practicing yoga, you really do not have to be flexible. As a matter of fact, yoga will help you become flexible. Since there are a lot of various yoga styles which range from gentle to vigorous, you may search for yoga instructor and style that will best suit your needs, class schedule, current physical condition, limitations and abilities.

Be sure that your instructor is aware of any health issues and your level of fitness. Do not force any poses or movements. Mastery of yoga poses will come with regular practice. Wear stretchable or lightly loose clothing that are comfortable. Expect to take off your shoes during a yoga session.

At the end of a yoga session, you must feel calm and invigorated and not in physical discomfort. Try attending yoga classes for twice a week or even more. A single yoga session typically lasts for about 60 minutes.

Following are some tips for yoga beginners:

1. Select a particular yoga type

   This step involves doing a little research on your part. A lot of yoga classes are available out there, and you will be most likely to be disappointed if you pick a certain yoga type that does not suit your state of physical fitness and personality.

   Take a couple of minutes to read the overview of yoga as provided on the first chapter of this book. For majority of yoga starters, vinyasa or hatha yoga class will be the most suitable, depending on whether you would like to go for a fast or slow-paced class. Keep in mind that these are just basic yoga classes and you can always go for something more advanced or fancier later.

2. Look for a yoga class

Try looking for yoga classes available in your locality. You may look at online resources, local alternative newspapers as well as wellness and fitness magazines for listings.

Go for a yoga studio that is convenient to your work or home so that it would be easy for you to get into class. Be sure to begin with a basic level yoga class. A lot of fitness centers and gyms also offer yoga sessions – this is a great place to get started if you are already a gym member. Finding a competent yoga instructor will help you to stick with your yoga classes.

3. Know what to bring during yoga classes

During the first day of your yoga class, you will not have to bring a lot of stuff except for yourself and some breathable, comfortable clothing. Majority of yoga studious have yoga mats available for rental.

4. Know what to expect

In a usual yoga class, the participants put their yoga mats in a loose grid facing the front of the room. This is usually identifiable by the instructor's mat or a small altar. It is strongly advised not to line up your yoga mat precisely with one next to it since you and your co-yogi will require some space in some yoga spaces. The participants usually sit in a cross-legged position.

The yoga instructor may commence the class by leading the class in reciting the syllable "om" thrice. Depending on the instructor, there could be some short meditation or some breathing exercises at the beginning of the session.

This is usually followed by warm-up yoga poses, then more vigorous poses. Next would be stretches and on to the final relaxation. If you need some rest at any time, take a child's pose.

Oftentimes, the instructor will roam around to every participant during the final relaxation and provide them with a little massage. Majority of yoga instructors end the session with another set of "oms".

The Do's and Don'ts during a Yoga Class

Do's:

- Familiarize yourself with some of starter's yoga poses before taking your first yoga session

- Ask the yoga instructor for help if you need it

- Inform your yoga instructor that it's going to be your first yoga session

- Review yoga etiquette so that you will feel very comfortable in a very unfamiliar situation

- Come back in a couple of days for your next yoga session

Don'ts:

- Wear socks or shoes during yoga sessions

- Drink water during the session, although have some before and after the class

- Have a good meal right before a yoga session. Try to eat light a couple of hours before the session begins

Conclusion

Now you have started your journey towards a better, yoga life. There will still be times when you struggle, and that is absolutely fine.

Like everything else in life – it's all about practice. The more you practice, the more you will be able to think just a little more rationally, which will help diffuse some of your stress immediately. Eventually you will get to a point where you can channel any bad energies around you into your weekly/daily yoga session without even pausing – but you likely are not there yet. Keep practicing, keep breathing, and don't forget to center yourself.

These techniques will help you with everything from climbing up the stairs to calming down before doing a big presentation. Remember that what you put into your body, you will get out of it. Don't stop moving, don't stop pushing the limits of your body, and don't forget that you can control your happiness and state of mind.

"When you drive around the city and come to a red light or a stop sign, you can just sit back and make use of these twenty or thirty seconds to relax — to breathe in, breathe out, and enjoy arriving in the present moment. There are many things like that we can do." **- Thich Nhat Hanh.**